THE SUGAR-FREE COOKBOOK

WILLIAM I. KAUFMAN is a native New Yorker whose hobby of cooking international dishes led him to writing cookbooks himself. Among these are *The Art of Creole Cookery, The Art of India's Cookery*, a four-volume series entitled *The Wonderful World of Cooking* and, forthcoming, *The Coffee Cookbook*, and *The Nut Cookbook*.

Mr. Kaufman has also traveled extensively and written several books on travel as well as on television in which he was an executive for sixteen years.

DEMETRIA TAYLOR, who supervised the kitchen testing of the recipes in this book, is a well-known consultant in the food field. She has been head of *McCall's* Kitchen, has been associated with *Good Housekeeping* Institute, has taught home economics, and is a member of the American Home Economics Association and the American Dietetic Association.

THE
SUGAR-FREE
COOKBOOK

By

WILLIAM I. KAUFMAN

Recipes Kitchen Tested by
DEMETRIA TAYLOR

Dolphin Books
DOUBLEDAY & COMPANY, INC.
Garden City, New York

The Dolphin Handbook edition is the first publication of
THE SUGAR-FREE COOKBOOK

Dolphin Books edition: 1964

Library of Congress Catalog Card Number 64–15774

CONTENTS

INTRODUCTION

If cutting down on sugar or cutting sugar out of your diet has been a problem, THE SUGAR-FREE COOKBOOK is for you! It has been created to introduce you to the use of a liquid no-calorie concentrated sweetener as a substitute for refined sugar in preparing the foods you like best so you can indulge your sweet tooth while watching your waistline or your health.

With the use of these sweeteners almost anyone can enjoy dishes that ordinarily call for sugar as an ingredient. Sweet syrups and savory sauces can be made. The salad eater may enjoy that glorious greenery with his favorite dressing. The dessert lover can indulge his fancy in the sweetest, richest, confectionery delights.

Modern science has perfected all manner of convenience foods to help out today's homemaker, but liquid no-calorie concentrated sweetener is not only easy to use, it enables the busy cook to satisfy many diet requirements without either making special dishes only for the dieter or compromising on taste, appearance, or dining pleasure for the whole family.

Traditionally, sweets and sweet tastes have been synonymous with happy times and special occasions. However, those who are on a restricted sugar regime often feel particularly limited at such celebrations. Through the use of the liquid no-calorie concentrated sweetener, the sweet taste is still there and the pleasures that go with it; all that's missing is the sugar.

Reminder to dieters: The natural sugars found in fruits and vegetables as well as the small quantities of refined sugar in prepared products such as ketchup, Kitchen Bouquet, Tabasco, and Worcestershire sauces should not be overlooked when you are planning your menus.

RULES FOR COOKING WITH LIQUID NO-CALORIE CONCENTRATED SWEETENERS

The recipes in this book have all been kitchen tested because there are many dishes in which no sugar substitute can be used successfully. For the sake of consistency, all these recipes were tested with Sweeta® liquid concentrated sweetener. The sugar calories replaced by sweetener are noted in each recipe so you may use any brand of sweetener by following its manufacturer's directions for sugar equivalents. Be sure to check these equivalents before you begin to cook.

There are three types of liquid, granular or tablet sweeteners: the cyclamate formula, the saccharine formula, and a formula of cyclamate and saccharine combined. Because of the individual differences in these formulas, proceed with caution when making substitutions, even in dishes you have previously cooked successfully with another sweetener.

Special Hints

1. Follow manufacturers' equivalency directions precisely. Concentrated liquid sweeteners vary in strength among themselves, and one drop too much of any formula can change a recipe.
2. It is suggested that you taste before adding the entire amount of sweetener ingredient called for by the recipe.
3. Whenever you have a choice, use the liquid concentrated sweetener at the end of the cooking process. This will enable you to test most accurately for sweetness.
4. The sweetening quality of any liquid concentrated sweetener tends to be accentuated by the addition of heat. It is better for this reason to add the sweetener after a dish has been removed from the heat. In any case, bear this in mind if you are planning to cook a dish ahead.
5. The sweetening quality of the liquid sweetener tends to be diminished by chilling or freezing.

MAIN DISHES

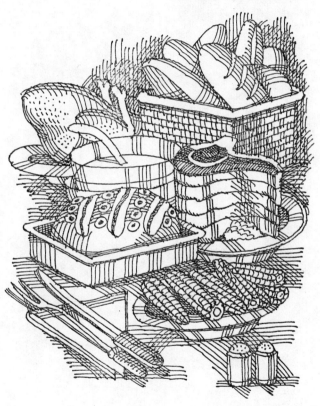

LAMB IN CURRY SAUCE

3 pounds boneless lamb, cubed
2 teaspoons salt
¼ teaspoon pepper
3 medium onions, finely chopped
2 tablespoons vegetable oil
1 tablespoon curry powder
¼ cup finely diced, peeled apple
1 cup cider vinegar
10 drops liquid concentrated sweetener
   (= 5 teaspoons sugar)
2 tablespoons cornstarch
1¼ cups water, divided

Sprinkle lamb evenly with salt and pepper. Sauté onions in oil until golden brown. Combine curry powder, apple, and vinegar; add to onions; simmer about 7 minutes. Remove from heat; stir in liquid sweetener; cool. Pour curry sauce over lamb; refrigerate overnight. Remove meat to shallow pan; broil, with surface of meat 4 inches below heat, for 30 minutes, stirring occasionally. Reheat curry sauce. Blend cornstarch with ¼ cup water; add to curry sauce with remaining water. Cook and stir until thickened. Simmer 10 minutes. Pour over broiled lamb. Serve with rice. Makes 6 servings. (*Calorie Savings: approximately 90*)

Kenny's Steak Pub, New York, New York

* BE SURE TO CHECK YOUR BRAND
OF SWEETENER'S SUGAR EQUIVALENT.

BRAISED DUCK GRENOBLE

2 tablespoons shortening
1 teaspoon Kitchen Bouquet
2 ducklings (3½ pounds each) quartered
1 can (12½ ounces) clear chicken broth
1 can dietetic Queen Anne cherries
½ cup port wine
¼ teaspoon salt
1 tablespoon cornstarch
12 drops liquid concentrated sweetener
    (= 2 tablespoons sugar)

Blend shortening and Kitchen Bouquet until creamy; brush evenly on ducklings. Place ducklings in large roasting pan. Roast at 325° for 1½ hours or until done. (After ½ hour pierce skin surfaces with tines of fork.) Remove ducklings to platter; keep warm. Pour fat from roasting pan, leaving only the brown drippings. Add chicken broth to roasting pan, reserving ¼ cup. Add cherries with their liquid, wine, and salt. Bring to a boil. Blend cornstarch with reserved chicken broth; add. Stir until sauce is thickened. Stir in liquid concentrated sweetener. Pour some of the sauce over duckling; serve the rest separately. Makes 8 servings. (*Calorie Savings: approximately 108*)

The Quorum Restaurant, Denver, Colorado

PEPPER STEAKS

1½ teaspoons crushed black pepper
  6 cube steaks (4 ounces each)
    Flour
¼ cup vegetable oil
  1 small onion, chopped
  1 small green pepper, cut in ½-inch squares
¼ cup flour
2½ cups water or bouillon
½ teaspoon salt
    Few grains nutmeg
  2 tablespoons dry sherry
 20 drops liquid concentrated sweetener
    (= 10 teaspoons sugar)
¼ cup tomato sauce
  1 pimiento, diced

Press black pepper evenly on both sides of steaks; dust with flour; brown on both sides in oil; remove from pan. Add onion and green pepper to pan; cook gently until tender. Stir in flour; brown lightly. Add water or bouillon; cook and stir until thickened; simmer 10 minutes. Stir in salt, nutmeg, sherry, sweetener, and tomato sauce; mix well. Return steaks to sauce; add pimiento; heat to serving temperature. Makes 4 servings. (*Calorie Savings: approximately 180*)

Nisi's Sparetime Cafe, Omaha, Nebraska

* BE SURE TO CHECK YOUR BRAND
OF SWEETENER'S SUGAR EQUIVALENT.

CHICKEN CAPER

     2 to 3 garlic cloves, crushed
     6 peppercorns
  2½ teaspoons oregano
     4 teaspoons salt
     1 tablespoon vinegar
     2 broiler-fryers, quartered
     6 large prunes, pitted
     8 small whole onions
     2 bay leaves
     6 green olives, pitted
     1 tablespoon capers
  1½ teaspoons liquid from jar of capers
     1 cup chicken stock or broth
   ¼ cup dry white wine
   10 drops liquid concentrated sweetener
        (= 5 teaspoons sugar)

Grind garlic, peppercorns, oregano, and salt with mortar
and pestle or crush with rolling pin; add vinegar; rub into
chicken pieces. Place chicken in deep skillet or Dutch oven.
Place prunes, onions, bay leaves, olives, capers, and caper
juice on top of chicken. Cover; chill overnight. Add chicken
broth. Bring to boil; reduce heat to medium; cook 10 minutes. Reduce heat to simmer; cook 1 hour. Add wine and
sweetener; simmer ½ hour longer. Makes 4 servings. (*Calorie Savings: approximately 90*)

CRANBERRY PORK CHOPS

6 *pork chops, cut 1-inch thick*
¼ *cup flour*
1 *teaspoon salt*
2 *tablespoons shortening*
2 *cups fresh cranberries*
1 *cup water*
1 *teaspoon liquid concentrated sweetener*
    (= *2 cups sugar*)

Dredge chops with flour and salt. Brown on both sides in shortening. Place chops in single layer in baking pan; pour cranberries over chops. Combine water and sweetener; pour over all. Cover pan (if no cover use aluminum foil). Bake at 350° for 30 minutes. Remove cover; bake 30 minutes longer or until chops are done. Makes 6 servings. (*Calorie Savings: approximately 1728*)

Cross Keys Restaurant, Fort Worth, Texas

* BE SURE TO CHECK YOUR BRAND
OF SWEETENER'S SUGAR EQUIVALENT.

OLD-STYLE POT ROAST

2 *tablespoons flour*
1 *tablespoon salt*
4 *pounds beef rump, round or chuck*
2 *tablespoons vegetable oil*
2 *carrots, diced*
1 *onion, sliced*
1 *tablespoon Worcestershire sauce*
½ *teaspoon nutmeg*
1 *cup water*
8 *drops liquid concentrated sweetener*
  (= *4 teaspoons sugar*)

Combine flour and salt; dredge beef with this mixture. Brown on all sides in vegetable oil. Add all remaining ingredients. Cover; simmer about 3½ hours or until beef is tender. Remove meat. Strain liquid in pan; reheat; serve with beef. (*Calorie Savings: approximately 72*)

Kenny's Steak Pub, New York, New York

CHICKEN MARIA

1 broiler-fryer chicken (3 pounds), disjointed
Salt and pepper
½ cup vegetable oil
¼ cup lemon juice
8 drops liquid concentrated sweetener
  (= 4 teaspoons sugar)
1 teaspoon oregano
1 cup dietetic canned tomatoes
Peel of 1 lemon

Sprinkle chicken pieces with salt and pepper. Combine oil, lemon juice, sweetener, and oregano; pour over chicken; marinate 1 hour, turning chicken occasionally. Remove chicken to baking pan; pour marinade mixture over chicken. Pour tomatoes over all. Top with thinly sliced lemon peel. Bake at 350° for 1½ hours, turning chicken pieces occasionally. Makes 4 servings. (*Calorie Savings: approximately 72*)

Rocky's White Shutter Inn, Des Moines, Iowa

* BE SURE TO CHECK YOUR BRAND
OF SWEETENER'S SUGAR EQUIVALENT.

LAMB AND TOMATO RAGOUT

2 tablespoons vegetable oil
2 medium onions, finely chopped
2 pounds boned lamb, cut in ½-inch cubes
8 small tomatoes, peeled and chopped
½ small hot red pepper, minced (optional)
8 drops liquid concentrated sweetener
  (= 4 teaspoons sugar)
  Salt and pepper to taste

Heat vegetable oil in heavy skillet or Dutch oven. Cook onions in oil until lightly browned. Add lamb; cook and stir until browned. Add tomatoes and red pepper. Cover. Simmer 2½ to 3 hours. Add sweetener, salt and pepper. Serve with rice. Makes 4 to 6 servings. (*Calorie Savings: approximately 72*)

Kenny's Steak Pub, New York, New York

BRAISED PORK BUTT

    1 boned, smoked pork butt, about 3 pounds
    ¾ cup soy sauce
    12 drops liquid concentrated sweetener
        (= 2 tablespoons sugar)
    1½ cups water
    1 tablespoon dry sherry
    2 stalks Chinese cabbage (optional)

Remove net covering from pork butt. Cut several gashes
½-inch deep in surface. Combine soy sauce, sweetener, water, and sherry; pour over meat. Simmer 2 hours, or until
meat is very tender, turning several times and adding more
water if sauce gets too thick. Cut up cabbage; add; cook
about 10 minutes on higher heat, or until cabbage is crisp-
tender. (Calorie Savings: approximately 108)

Shanghai East Restaurant, New York, New York

* BE SURE TO CHECK YOUR BRAND
OF SWEETENER'S SUGAR EQUIVALENT.

[23]

MOCK HAM LOAF WITH CUMBERLAND SAUCE

1½ *pounds top round, ground*
1 *cup quick-cooking rolled oats*
1½ *cups tomato juice, divided*
2 *eggs*
¼ *teaspoon liquid concentrated sweetener*
 (= ½ cup sugar)
¼ *teaspoon liquid smoke*
1 *teaspoon salt*
1 *teaspoon minced onion*
1 *tablespoon butter*
1 *teaspoon cornstarch*
½ *cup water*
2 *drops liquid concentrated sweetener*
 (= 1 teaspoon sugar)

Combine meat, oats, 1 cup tomato juice, eggs, ¼ teaspoon sweetener, liquid smoke, and salt. Mix thoroughly. Pack into well-greased loaf pan, 7½ × 3½ × 2½ inches. Bake at 350° for 1 hour. Pour off juice into saucepan. Add remaining tomato juice, onion, and butter. Heat and stir until butter melts and onion is soft. Blend cornstarch with a little of the water; add remaining water; add to saucepan. Cook and stir until slightly thickened; simmer 10 minutes longer. Add 2 drops sweetener. Serve with meat loaf. Makes 6 to 8 servings. (*Calorie Savings: approximately 500*)

Nisi's Sparetime Cafe, Omaha, Nebraska

SPAGHETTI WITH SCALLOP SAUCE

    1 large onion, chopped (1 cup)
    ½ clove garlic, minced
    1 tablespoon olive oil
    1 can (1 pound) dietetic tomatoes
    1 can (6 ounces) tomato paste
    ½ cup water
    ¼ cup chopped parsley
    1 tablespoon mixed Italian herbs
 1½ teaspoons salt
    ¼ teaspoon pepper
    1 pound fresh sea scallops, washed and chopped
    4 drops liquid concentrated sweetener
      (= 2 teaspoons sugar)
    1 package (1 pound) thin spaghetti, cooked and
      drained
      Grated Parmesan cheese

Sauté onion and garlic in olive oil in large saucepan just until softened. Stir in tomatoes, tomato paste, water, parsley, Italian herbs, salt and pepper. Cover; simmer 1 hour. Stir in scallops and sweetener; cook 15 minutes longer, or until scallops are tender. Spoon over spaghetti, or toss with spaghetti just before serving; pass cheese separately to sprinkle over. Makes 6 servings. (*Calorie Savings: approximately 36*)

Riviera Restaurant, Atlanta, Georgia

* BE SURE TO CHECK YOUR BRAND
OF SWEETENER'S SUGAR EQUIVALENT.

BARBECUED BEEF PATTIES

        1 cup soft bread crumbs
     ½ cup milk
        1 pound lean beef, ground
        1 teaspoon salt
           Few grains pepper
    4½ teaspoons Worcestershire sauce
     ¼ cup vinegar
        8 drops liquid concentrated sweetener
           (= 4 teaspoons sugar)
     ½ cup ketchup
     ½ cup chopped green pepper
        2 tablespoons minced onion

Combine bread crumbs and milk; let stand 5 minutes. Combine soaked crumbs, beef, salt and pepper. Shape into 8 patties; place in baking dish. Combine remaining ingredients; pour around patties. Bake at 375° for 45 minutes. Makes 4 servings. (*Calorie Savings: approximately 72*)

Kenny's Steak Pub, New York, New York

DUCKLING WITH TANGERINES

3 *large tangerines*
1 *duckling (3½ pounds), quartered*
2 *cups chicken broth*
1 *tablespoon cornstarch*
1 *tablespoon lemon juice*
12 *drops liquid concentrated sweetener*
   (= *2 tablespoons sugar*)

Grate peel of 1 tangerine; set aside. Place duckling in roasting pan; add chicken broth. Bake at 325° for 2 hours, or until duckling is very tender. Remove duckling. Pour off all but 3 tablespoons of pan drippings. Squeeze all 3 tangerines; measure juice; if necessary, add enough water (or orange juice) to make 1 cup; add to pan. Blend cornstarch and lemon juice; stir into liquid in pan. Cook and stir until thickened and clear. Remove from heat; stir in sweetener and grated peel. Pour over duckling. Makes 4 servings. (*Calorie Savings: approximately 108*)

Hotel Westward Ho, Phoenix, Arizona

* BE SURE TO CHECK YOUR BRAND
OF SWEETENER'S SUGAR EQUIVALENT.

[27]

VEGETABLES

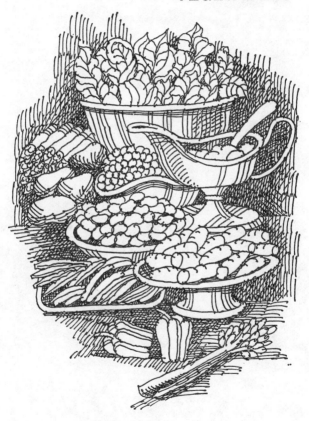

FRESH ASPARAGUS WITH HOT BACON DRESSING

¼ *pound sliced bacon*
2 *white onions, finely chopped*
¼ *cup vinegar*
¼ *cup water*
    Salt to taste
6 *drops liquid concentrated sweetener*
    (= *1 tablespoon sugar*)
1 *large bunch fresh asparagus* or
2 *packages (10 ounces each) frozen*
    asparagus, cooked

Dice bacon fine; cook in skillet until crisp. Add onions; cook until tender. Add vinegar, water, and salt. Bring to a boil. Remove from heat; stir in sweetener; pour over hot asparagus. Makes 6 servings. (*Calorie Savings: approximately 54*)

The Occidental, Washington, D.C.

* BE SURE TO CHECK YOUR BRAND
OF SWEETENER'S SUGAR EQUIVALENT.

[31]

TOMATOES VINAIGRETTE

Empty 2 cans (1 pound each) peeled whole tomatoes. Carefully lift out tomatoes and place in serving dish or individual bowls. (Serve juice as a beverage or use in soup or stew.) Measure 2 tablespoons vinegar into a cup; stir in 3 drops liquid concentrated sweetener (= *1½ teaspoons sugar*). Spoon over tomatoes; sprinkle lightly with salt and pepper, then with ½ teaspoon dried dill weed. Garnish with onion rings. Chill. Makes 6 servings. (*Calorie Savings: approximately 27*)

Jacques' Restaurant, Chicago, Illinois

ACORN SQUASH WITH PINEAPPLE

2 acorn squash
4 teaspoons butter or margarine
2 tablespoons dry sherry
¼ teaspoon nutmeg
½ teaspoon salt
½ cup finely chopped fresh or
   dietetic canned pineapple
14 drops liquid concentrated sweetener
   (= 7 teaspoons sugar)

Cut squash in half lengthwise; scoop out stringy pulp and seeds. Pour water into baking pan to a depth of ½ inch. Place squash, cut side down in baking pan. Bake at 400° for 20 minutes. Turn cut side up. Dot with butter and sprinkle with half the sherry. Bake 25 minutes longer, or until squash is tender. Remove squash from pan; scoop out pulp; combine pulp with remaining ingredients; blend well. Refill shells. Empty water from baking pan; replace squash in pan, cut side up. Bake 10 minutes longer. Makes 4 servings. (*Calorie Savings: approximately 126*)

The Quorum Restaurant, Denver, Colorado

* BE SURE TO CHECK YOUR BRAND
OF SWEETENER'S SUGAR EQUIVALENT.

CANDIED YAMS

½ *cup butter or margarine*
1⅓ *cups water*
½ *teaspoon liquid concentrated sweetener*
  (*= 1 cup sugar*)
½ *teaspoon cinnamon*
½ *teaspoon nutmeg*
 4 *large yams, cooked and sliced*
 3 *teaspoons coarsely grated orange peel*

Combine butter, water, sweetener, and spices; heat until butter melts. Arrange a layer of sliced yams (about ⅓) in shallow, greased baking pan. Pour ⅓ butter mixture over them. Scatter 1 teaspoon orange peel over top. Repeat until all ingredients are used. Bake at 350° for about 30 minutes. Makes 6 servings. (*Calorie Savings: approximately 864*)

Smith's Cross Lake Inn, Shreveport, Louisiana

DILL MUSHROOMS

 2 *cans (3 or 4 ounces each) whole mushrooms*
½ *cup white vinegar*
 8 *drops liquid concentrated sweetener*
  (*= 4 teaspoons sugar*)
 1 *teaspoon salt*
½ *teaspoon dried dill weed*

Pour mushrooms and liquid into small bowl; add vinegar, sweetener, salt, and dill weed; mix well; cover. Chill several hours or overnight to blend seasonings; drain before serving. Makes 6 servings. (*Calorie Savings: approximately 72*)

VEGETABLE RELISH

3 cups finely chopped cabbage
1 medium-size cucumber, pared and chopped
½ cup chopped green pepper
2 pimientos, chopped
6 drops liquid concentrated sweetener
  (= 1 tablespoon sugar)
1 teaspoon salt
1 tablespoon lemon juice
1 tablespoon water

Combine cabbage, cucumber, green pepper, and pimientos. Mix remaining ingredients; pour over vegetables; toss to mix. Cover; chill. Makes 4 servings. (*Calorie Savings: approximately 54*)

Trinkaus Manor, Orsikany, New York

* BE SURE TO CHECK YOUR BRAND
OF SWEETENER'S SUGAR EQUIVALENT.

SALADS
AND
SALAD DRESSINGS

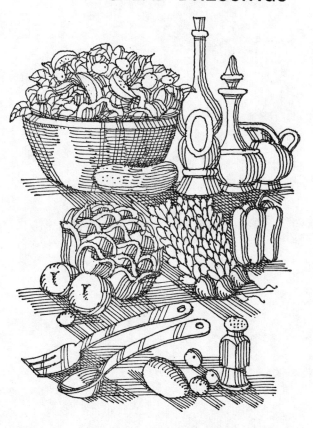

SWEET SEASONED VINEGAR

1 cup cider vinegar
1 teaspoon liquid concentrated sweetener
 (= 2 cups sugar)
1 tablespoon salt
1 teaspoon black pepper

Combine all ingredients; mix well. Makes about 1 cup.
(*Calorie Savings: approximately 1728*)

Miss Hulling's Cafeterias, St. Louis, Missouri

SPANISH SLAW

1 quart shredded cabbage
1 tablespoon salad oil
2 tablespoons chopped pimiento
¼ cup chopped green pepper
1 tablespoon chopped onion
½ cup Sweet Seasoned Vinegar (see recipe above)

Mix cabbage and oil until cabbage is coated with oil. Add
pimiento, pepper, and onion; toss to combine thoroughly.
Add Sweet Seasoned Vinegar. Mix and serve. Makes 4
servings. (*Calorie Savings: approximtaely 864*)

Miss Hulling's Cafeterias, St. Louis, Missouri

* BE SURE TO CHECK YOUR BRAND
OF SWEETENER'S SUGAR EQUIVALENT.

HOLIDAY CRANBERRY SALAD

4 cups fresh cranberries
2 cups boiling water
1 teaspoon liquid concentrated sweetener
  (= 2 cups sugar)
  Juice of 1 orange
3 tablespoons unflavored gelatine
½ cup cold water
1 red apple
1 cup finely sliced celery
1 cup chopped walnuts

Cook cranberries in boiling water for about 10 minutes, or until skins pop; put through food mill or sieve. Stir in sweetener and orange juice. Soften gelatine in cold water; add to hot, sieved cranberries; stir until dissolved. Chill until slightly thickened. Meanwhile, dice unpeeled red apple; combine with celery and walnuts; fold into gelatine mixture. Spoon into 5-cup mold. Chill until set. Unmold on crisp salad greens. Serve with dietetic mayonnaise. Makes 8 to 10 servings. (*Calorie Savings: approximately 1728*)

Tubbert's Restaurant, Syracuse, New York

WILTED SALAD

    2 heads Bibb lettuce*
 ½ pound bacon, diced
    1 teaspoon Worcestershire sauce
    6 drops Tabasco
 ¼ cup wine vinegar
 ¼ teaspoon salt
    8 drops liquid concentrated sweetener
       (= 4 teaspoons sugar)

Wash lettuce; separate leaves. Cook diced bacon until crisp. Add remaining ingredients to bacon and bacon fat; bring to a boil; pour over lettuce; reduce heat to low for about 3 minutes, to wilt lettuce. Makes 4 servings. (*Calorie Savings: approximately 72*)

* Other types of lettuce may be used, if desired.

The Windsor Restaurant, Los Angeles, California

* BE SURE TO CHECK YOUR BRAND
OF SWEETENER'S SUGAR EQUIVALENT.

LOW-CALORIE SALAD DRESSING

   1 garlic clove, minced
   ¼ cup vinegar
   ½ cup orange juice
   ¼ teaspoon paprika
   5 drops liquid concentrated sweetener
       (= 2½ teaspoons sugar)
   ½ teaspoon salt
   ⅛ teaspoon pepper

Add garlic to vinegar; let stand 1 hour; strain. Add remaining ingredients to garlic-vinegar; shake well. Chill. Shake again before using. Makes about ¾ cup. (*Calorie Savings: approximately 45*)

Tony and Luigi's, Lincoln, Nebraska

SWEET HERB DRESSING

   1 cup vegetable oil
   2 cups cider vinegar
  25 drops liquid concentrated sweetener
       (= 12½ teaspoons sugar)
   1 teaspoon salt
   ½ teaspoon sweet basil
   2 tablespoons minced onion
   2 garlic cloves, crushed
   1 tablespoon chopped parsley

Combine all ingredients; shake well. Makes about 3 cups. Beat with rotary beater before serving. (*Calorie Savings: approximately 225*)

Corn Husker Hotel, Lincoln, Nebraska

BEAN SALAD TRIO

1 can (1 pound) green beans
1 can (1 pound) wax beans
1 can (1 pound) kidney beans
½ cup vinegar
¼ teaspoon liquid concentrated sweetener
    (= ½ cup sugar)
¼ cup vegetable oil
¼ cup chopped onion
½ cup sliced celery
½ teaspoon oregano
½ teaspoon tarragon

Drain and combine green, wax, and kidney beans; combine remaining ingredients; mix well; pour over bean mixture; mix well. Chill several hours. Serve on crisp salad greens with dietetic mayonnaise, if desired. Makes 6 to 8 servings. (*Calorie Savings: approximately 432*)

Doc's Air Park Restaurant, Quincy, Illinois

* BE SURE TO CHECK YOUR BRAND
OF SWEETENER'S SUGAR EQUIVALENT.

SWEET-SOUR SALAD DRESSING

1 green pepper
1 medium onion
1 can (8 ounces) tomato sauce
½ teaspoon liquid concentrated sweetener
    (= 1 cup sugar)
1 cup vinegar
1 cup vegetable oil
1 teaspoon salt
1 teaspoon monosodium glutamate

Put green pepper and onion through food chopper using fine knife. Combine with remaining ingredients; mix thoroughly. Makes about 1 quart. (*Calorie Savings: approximately 864*)

Doc's Air Park Restaurant, Quincy, Illinois

SOUR-CREAM SALAD DRESSING

1 cup dairy sour cream
2 tablespoons white vinegar
1 teaspoon salt
¼ teaspoon liquid concentrated sweetener
*   (= ½ cup sugar)*
3 tablespoons cold water
Few grains white pepper

Combine all ingredients; mix well. Makes 4 servings. Excellent for cole slaw, sliced cucumbers, or Belgian endive. (*Calorie Savings: approximately 432*)

University Club, San Antonio, Texas

WILTED SPINACH SALAD

1 pound fresh spinach
2 tablespoons lemon juice
1 teaspoon vegetable oil
¼ teaspoon seasoned salt
¼ teaspoon Worcestershire sauce
2 drops liquid concentrated sweetener
*   (= 1 teaspoon sugar)*

Cut out any large ribs and all stems from spinach; wash leaves well; drain. Steam, covered, in large saucepan, without adding any water, 2 to 3 minutes, or just until wilted. Drain. Combine remaining ingredients in cup; pour over spinach; toss to coat leaves well. Spoon into heated serving dish. Makes 6 servings. (*Calorie Savings: approximately 18*)

Riviera Restaurant, Atlanta, Georgia

* BE SURE TO CHECK YOUR BRAND
OF SWEETENER'S SUGAR EQUIVALENT.

JULIENNE SALAD WITH A SWEET-SOUR DRESSING

>   1 head leaf lettuce
>   ¼ pound cooked ham, cut in Julienne strips
>   ¼ pound sharp cheddar cheese, cut in Julienne strips
>   2 tablespoons cut chives
>   2 tablespoons chopped parsley
>   4 raw mushrooms, sliced through stem
>   ½ cup vegetable oil
>   ½ cup wine vinegar
>   ¼ teaspoon liquid concentrated sweetener
>   (= ½ cup sugar)
>   Few grains pepper
>   1 teaspoon dry mustard

Arrange lettuce in salad bowl. Top with ham, cheese, chives, parsley, and mushrooms. Combine remaining ingredients; mix well; pour over salad. Toss to mix. Makes 4 servings. (*Calorie Savings: approximately 432*)

University Club, San Antonio, Texas

KIDNEY BEANS VINAIGRETTE

>   1 can (1 pound) red kidney beans, drained
>   ¼ cup chopped Spanish onion
>   ¼ cup diced green pepper
>   ½ cup finely sliced celery
>   2 tablespoons chopped pimiento
>   ¼ cup Sweet Seasoned Vinegar (see page 39)
>   1 tablespoon salad oil

Combine all ingredients; chill. Makes 6 servings. (*Calorie Savings: approximately 432*)

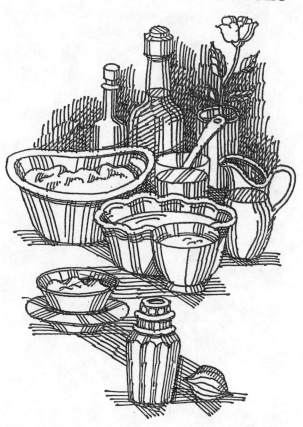

SAUCES

DILL SAUCE
(for boiled lamb or beef)

    3 tablespoons butter or margarine
    3 tablespoons flour
 1½ cups hot meat stock
  ½ cup milk
    3 tablespoons chopped fresh dill or
      3 teaspoons dried dill weed
    2 tablespoons vinegar
    4 drops liquid concentrated sweetener
      (= 2 teaspoons sugar)
      Salt to taste
    1 egg, slightly beaten

Melt butter; blend in flour. Combine stock, milk, and dill; stir in gradually. Cook and stir over medium heat until smooth and thickened; simmer 10 minutes. Add vinegar, sweetener, and salt. Pour a little of the hot sauce on egg; return to remaining sauce; blend. Heat, stirring, for 1 minute (do not boil). Makes about 2 cups. (*Calorie Savings: approximately 36*)

* BE SURE TO CHECK YOUR BRAND
OF SWEETENER'S SUGAR EQUIVALENT.

BARBECUE SAUCE
(for any kind of meat or poultry)

½ cup red wine vinegar
½ cup vegetable oil
1 cup dry red wine
3 cloves garlic
2 bay leaves, crumbled
½ teaspoon rosemary
½ teaspoon liquid concentrated sweetener
   (= 1 cup sugar)
½ teaspoon salt
½ teaspoon freshly ground pepper
6 whole cloves
1 medium onion, finely grated
1 teaspoon chopped parsley
1 tablespoon soy sauce

Combine all ingredients, stir or beat until well blended. Makes 3 cups. (*Calorie Savings: approximately 864*)

To use: place meat in pan; pour sauce over it. Chill 4 to 12 hours. When ready to use drain meat; place on grill. Reserve sauce. Baste meat frequently with sauce while broiling.

University Club, San Antonio, Texas

CREOLE SAUCE

1 medium green pepper, diced
2 stalks celery, sliced thin
1 medium onion, chopped
1 can (3 or 4 ounces) sliced mushrooms
1 can (1 pound) tomatoes
1 teaspoon salt
¼ teaspoon pepper
4 drops liquid concentrated sweetener
    (= 2 teaspoons sugar)

Combine all ingredients except sweetener; simmer 30 to 35 minutes. Add sweetener; mix well; remove from heat. Serve over rice, chicken, or vegetables. Makes 4 to 6 servings. (*Calorie Savings: approximately 36*)

Aldino's Manor, Wilkes-Barre, Pennsylvania

* BE SURE TO CHECK YOUR BRAND
OF SWEETENER'S SUGAR EQUIVALENT.

HOLIDAY FRUIT SAUCE FOR HAM STEAK

½ cup seedless raisins
2 cups hot water
1 cup orange juice or
  Unsweetened pineapple juice
⅛ teaspoon ground cloves
2 tablespoons cornstarch
¼ cup cold water
½ teaspoon liquid concentrated sweetener
  (= 1 cup sugar)

Cover raisins with hot water; let stand until raisins are plumped. Add fruit juice; bring to boil; simmer 2 minutes. Combine cloves and cornstarch; blend with ¼ cup cold water; add to sauce. Cook and stir until thickened and clear; simmer 10 minutes longer. Stir in sweetener. Makes about 2½ cups. (*Calorie Savings: approximately 864*)

The Inn At The Landing, Kansas City, Missouri

GOLDEN SAUCE

Beat 2 egg yolks with 1 cup skim milk and 18 drops liquid concentrated sweetener (= *3 tablespoons sugar*) until blended in top of double boiler. Cook, stirring constantly, over simmering water, 10 minutes, or until mixture coats spoon; remove from heat. Stir in 1 teaspoon vanilla and ¼ teaspoon lemon extract; serve warm. Makes 1¼ cups. (*Calorie Savings: approximately 162*)

Henry's, Cherry Hill, New Jersey

LEMON SAUCE FOR PUDDINGS

    2 *tablespoons cornstarch*
    2 *teaspoons grated lemon peel*
    2 *cups water*
    ½ *teaspoon liquid concentrated sweetener*
        (= *1 cup sugar*)
    ¼ *cup lemon juice*
    4 *tablespoons butter or margarine*
    ¼ *teaspoon salt*

Mix cornstarch and lemon peel in top of double boiler. Add water slowly; cook, stirring constantly, until thickened. Cook over hot water 10 minutes, stirring occasionally. Remove from heat; add sweetener, lemon juice, butter or margarine, and salt. Stir until butter melts. Makes 6 servings. (*Calorie Savings: approximately 864*)

* BE SURE TO CHECK YOUR BRAND
OF SWEETENER'S SUGAR EQUIVALENT.

STRAWBERRY FILLING OR TOPPING

2 cups (1 pint) strawberries, washed
1 cup water
2 tablespoons cornstarch
¼ teaspoon liquid concentrated sweetener
    (= ½ cup sugar)
1 teaspoon vanilla

Hull and slice berries. Stir water, a little at a time, into cornstarch until blended. Stir in sliced berries. Cook, stirring constantly and mashing berries well with back of spoon, over low heat until mixture thickens and boils 3 minutes. Remove from heat; stir in sweetener and vanilla; cool. Makes about 2 cups. (*Calorie Savings: approximately 432*)

La Tunisia, Dallas, Texas

GLAZE FOR FRUIT TARTS OR PIES

¾ cup unsweetened fruit juice (*orange, cherry, grape, berry, or any desired flavor*)
1 tablespoon cornstarch
15 drops liquid concentrated sweetener
    (= 7½ teaspoons sugar)

Add a little fruit juice to cornstarch; blend smooth; add remaining fruit juice. Cook and stir over hot (not boiling) water, until thick and clear. Remove from heat; stir in sweetener. Cool; pour over surface of fruit tarts or pie. Makes enough for 6 tarts or 1 pie. (*Calorie Savings: approximately 135*)

The Dogwood Room, Airport 77 Restaurant
Charlotte, North Carolina

CUSTARD

    2 cups milk
    3 egg yolks, slightly beaten
      Few grains salt
   12 drops (or to taste) liquid concentrated sweetener
      (= 2 tablespoons sugar)

Heat milk to scalding point. Pour slowly on egg yolks, stirring constantly. Stir in salt. Cook over hot (not boiling) water, stirring constantly, until mixture coats spoon. Stir in sweetener. Pour into serving dish; chill. Makes 6 servings. (*Calorie Savings: approximately 108*)

Martha Washington Inn, Abingdon, Virginia

WHIPPED TOPPING

   ¼ cup nonfat dry-milk solids
   ¼ cup cold water
    1 tablespoon lemon juice
    4 to 6 drops liquid concentrated sweetener
      (= 2–3 teaspoons sugar)

Combine dry milk and cold water; beat until soft peaks form. Add lemon juice; beat until stiff. Beat in sweetener. Makes 4 to 6 servings. (*Calorie Savings: approximately 36–54*)

* BE SURE TO CHECK YOUR BRAND
OF SWEETENER'S SUGAR EQUIVALENT.

DESSERTS

PETITE PARTY PUFFS

1½ cups water, divided
  3 tablespoons vegetable oil
  ½ cup flour
  ¾ teaspoon salt, divided
  2 eggs
  3 tablespoons cornstarch, divided
  2 tablespoons evaporated milk
  1 egg yolk, slightly beaten
 18 drops liquid concentrated sweetener
       (= 3 tablespoons sugar)
  1 teaspoon vanilla, divided
  ½ teaspoon lemon juice
  1 tablespoon butter or margarine
  2 tablespoons dietetic cocoa
  1 cup skim milk
  ½ teaspoon liquid concentrated sweetener
       (= 1 cup sugar)

Combine ½ cup water and vegetable oil in 1-quart sauce-pan; bring to boil. Add flour and ½ teaspoon salt; stir over medium heat until mixture leaves sides of pan and forms a ball around spoon. Remove from heat. Add eggs, one at a time, beating well after each addition. Drop from teaspoon onto well-greased baking sheet, spacing 1 inch apart, making 30 mounds. Bake at 400° for 25 to 30 minutes. Cool.

Combine 2 tablespoons cornstarch and remaining ¼ teaspoon salt in saucepan. Add remaining 1 cup water. Stir until smooth. Add evaporated milk. Cook and stir over medium heat until mixture comes to a boil and thickens. Add a little of this mixture to beaten egg yolk; return to saucepan; cook and stir about 2 minutes longer. Stir in 18

* BE SURE TO CHECK YOUR BRAND
OF SWEETENER'S SUGAR EQUIVALENT.

drops sweetener and ½ teaspoon vanilla. Cool slightly; stir in lemon juice. Chill.

Melt butter. Combine cocoa, remaining 1 tablespoon cornstarch, and a few grains additional salt; stir into melted butter. Add skim milk. Cook and stir over medium heat until thickened. Remove from heat; stir in remaining ½ teaspoon vanilla and ½ teaspoon sweetener. Cool.

To serve, slit puffs; fill with custard; top with chocolate sauce. Makes 10 servings of 3 puffs each. (*Calorie Savings: approximately 1026*)

Tubbert's Restaurant, Syracuse, New York

CUP CUSTARDS

    3 eggs
    ½ teaspoon grated lemon peel
    ⅛ teaspoon salt
    2¼ cups skim milk
    ½ teaspoon vanilla
    24 drops liquid concentrated sweetener
        (= ¼ cup sugar)

Beat eggs slightly with lemon peel and salt in medium-size bowl. Stir in milk, vanilla, and sweetener. Strain into 6 custard cups, using about ½ cup for each. Set cups in shallow pan; place on oven shelf; pour boiling water into pan to depth of 1 inch. Bake at 325° for 40 minutes, or until centers are almost set but still soft. (Custard will set as it cools.) Remove at once from pan of water. Serve warm or chilled, in cups, or unmold by first loosening custards around edges with a thin-blade knife, then inverting into serving dishes. Makes 6 servings. (*Calorie Savings: approximately 216*)

Columbia Restaurant, Tampa, Florida

CHOCO-CHIP PEAR VELVET

  1 egg, separated
  ½ cup water
     Dash of salt
  ¼ teaspoon liquid concentrated sweetener
     (= ½ cup sugar)
  1 envelope unflavored gelatine
  3 tablespoons instant nonfat dry milk
  1 teaspoon vanilla
  2 containers (8 ounces each) yogurt
  1 can (1 pound) dietetic quartered pears, drained
  1 tablespoon grated unsweetened chocolate

Beat egg yolk slightly; beat in water, salt, and sweetener.
Mix gelatine and dry milk in top of double boiler; stir in
egg-yolk mixture. Cook, stirring constantly, over simmering water, 5 minutes, or until gelatine dissolves and mixture
coats spoon. Strain into a large bowl; stir in vanilla. Chill
30 minutes, or just until mixture is as thick as unbeaten egg
white; blend in yogurt until creamy smooth. Beat egg white
until it forms soft peaks; fold into yogurt mixture. Pour
into a 4-cup shallow mold or an 8-inch layer-cake pan.
Chill 3 to 4 hours, or until firm. To unmold, run a sharp-tip,
thin-blade knife around top of mold, then dip mold very
quickly in and out of a pan of hot water. Invert on chilled
serving plate; lift off mold. Arrange pear quarters in a ring
on top; sprinkle with grated chocolate. Cut into wedges.
Makes 6 servings. (Calorie Savings: approximately 432)

The Cloud Room, Airport Terminal
Des Moines, Iowa

* BE SURE TO CHECK YOUR BRAND
OF SWEETENER'S SUGAR EQUIVALENT.

LOW-CALORIE COFFEE JELLY

2 envelopes unflavored gelatine
½ cup cold water
3½ cups freshly brewed strong coffee
32 drops liquid concentrated sweetener
    (= 16 teaspoons sugar)
½ teaspoon vanilla
    Dash of salt

Soften gelatine in cold water; add hot coffee; stir until gelatine dissolves; stir in sweetener, vanilla, and salt. Pour into shallow pan, 8 × 8 × 2 inches; chill 2 hours, or until firm. Break up with a fork. Spoon into 6 dessert dishes dividing evenly; top each with 1 tablespoon whipped cream, if desired. Makes 6 servings. (*Calorie Savings: approximately 288*)

Fan and Bill's Restaurant, Atlanta, Georgia

STRAWBERRIES MACIEL

3 tablespoons Jamaica rum
1 pint fresh strawberries
¾ cup orange juice
12 drops liquid concentrated sweetener
    (= 2 tablespoons sugar)
1 pint Vanilla Ice Cream (see page 68)

Sprinkle rum evenly over berries. Heat orange juice to a boil in chafing dish. Stir in sweetener. Add strawberries. Spoon over Vanilla Ice Cream. Makes 4 servings. (*Calorie Savings: approximately 108*)

Westport Room, A Fred Harvey Restaurant
Kansas City, Missouri

CUSTARD PIE

    4 *eggs*
 ¼ *teaspoon salt*
 ⅛ *teaspoon nutmeg*
    1 *teaspoon grated lemon peel*
    3 *cups skim milk*
 32 *drops liquid concentrated sweetener*
       (= *16 teaspoons sugar*)
    1 *teaspoon vanilla*
    1 *baked 9-inch pie shell*

Beat eggs slightly with salt, nutmeg, and lemon peel; stir in remaining ingredients. Set pie plate on a cookie sheet; place on rack in oven; strain custard mixture into prepared shell. Bake at 450° for 10 minutes; reduce heat to 300° and bake 45 minutes longer, or until center is almost set but still soft. (Do not overbake, for custard will set as it cools.) Cool pie on wire rack. Cut into 8 wedges. (*Calorie Savings: approximately 288*)

Weaver's Cafeteria, Knoxville, Tennessee

* BE SURE TO CHECK YOUR BRAND
OF SWEETENER'S SUGAR EQUIVALENT.

FOUNTAINS CREAM DELIGHT

1 envelope unflavored gelatine
¼ cup cold water
2 cups milk
⅛ teaspoon salt
3 eggs, separated
¼ teaspoon liquid concentrated sweetener
    (= ½ cup sugar)
1 teaspoon vanilla

Soften gelatine in cold water. Scald milk; add gelatine and salt; stir until gelatine dissolves. Beat egg yolks slightly; add a little of the hot-milk mixture slowly, while stirring; stir into remaining milk mixture. Cook and stir over hot (not boiling) water until slightly thickened. Add sweetener and vanilla; chill until mixture begins to congeal. Beat egg whites stiff; fold in. Spoon into individual molds; chill until firm. Unmold. Serve with any dietetic fruit. Makes 6 servings. (*Calorie Savings: approximately 432*)

The Fountains Restaurant, Binghamton, New York

PEACH CUSTARD PIE

    4 dietetic sliced peaches, drained
    1 unbaked 10-inch pie shell
    ⅓ cup grated fresh coconut (optional)
    4 eggs
    ½ teaspoon salt
    2 teaspoons vanilla
    ½ teaspoon liquid concentrated sweetener
        (= 1 cup sugar)
 2⅔ cups skim milk

Arrange peach slices in pie shell; scatter coconut over
peaches. Combine eggs, salt, vanilla, and sweetener; beat
until blended. Stir in milk; mix well; pour into pie shell.
Bake at 425° for about 40 minutes or until filling puffs up
and shakes like partially set gelatine. Chill. (*Calorie Savings: approximately 864*)

Hotel Lincoln Douglas, Quincy, Illinois

* BE SURE TO CHECK YOUR BRAND
OF SWEETENER'S SUGAR EQUIVALENT.

GRAPEFRUIT HALVES WITH KIRSCHWASSER

    2 grapefruit
    4 to 8 drops liquid concentrated sweetener, depend-
        ing on sweetness of grapefruit
        (= 2 to 4 teaspoons sugar)
    ¼ cup Kirschwasser

Halve grapefruit; separate each section from membrane, using sharp knife. Remove core and membrane, using scissors. Add sweetener to Kirschwasser; brush evenly over tops of grapefruit halves. Broil, with surface of fruit 3 to 4 inches below heat, until flecked with golden brown. Makes 4 servings. (*Calorie Savings: approximately 36 to 72*)

Brennan's, New Orleans, Louisiana

SWISS APPLE CUSTARD PIE

    3 cooking apples
    1 unbaked 9-inch pie shell
    2 cups milk, scalded
      Few grains salt
    ¼ teaspoon liquid concentrated sweetener
      (= ½ cup sugar)
    4 eggs, slightly beaten

Core and peel apples; cut in thin slices; arrange in pie shell. Bake at 425° for 12 minutes. Meanwhile, combine scalded milk, salt, and sweetener; pour slowly on beaten eggs; mix well. Remove pie from oven; lower heat to 350°. Pour milk mixture slowly over pie, waiting at intervals for milk to seep through apples. Bake at 350° for 40 minutes or until custard is set. (*Calorie Savings: approximately 432*)

Grison's Steak House, San Francisco, California

CINNAMON PEARS

Halve, core, and pare 4 medium-size, firm, ripe pears; place, cut side down, in large frying pan. Combine ½ cup water with 24 drops liquid concentrated sweetener (= ¼ *cup sugar*). Pour over pears; add 1 two-inch stick of cinnamon; cover pan. Heat to boiling; simmer 10 minutes, or just until pears are tender. Spoon into serving dish; pour any sauce from pan over pears. Serve warm or chilled. Makes 8 servings. (*Calorie Savings: approximately 216*)

Jacques' Restaurant, Chicago, Illinois

VANILLA FROZEN CUSTARD

   2 *envelopes unflavored gelatine*
   ½ *cup cold water*
   2 *cups instant nonfat dry-milk crystals*
   1 *quart whole milk*
   ½ *teaspoon liquid concentrated sweetener*
      (= *1 cup sugar*)
   2 *teaspoons vanilla*

Soften gelatine in cold water. Stir instant crystals into whole milk; blend in softened gelatine. Cook over low heat, stirring constantly, until gelatine dissolves. Cool. Stir in sweetener and vanilla. Turn into 2 refrigerator trays; freeze until firm; beat until smooth. Makes about 1 quart. (*Calorie Savings: approximately 864*)

Note: Best when served at once; texture changes on prolonged freezing.

Olde College Inn, Houston, Texas

* BE SURE TO CHECK YOUR BRAND
OF SWEETENER'S SUGAR EQUIVALENT.

VANILLA ICE CREAM

   1½ cups undiluted evaporated milk
   1 teaspoon unflavored gelatine
   2 tablespoons cold water
   1 cup skim milk
   1 tablespoon flour
   Few grains salt
   1 teaspoon liquid concentrated sweetener, divided
   (= 2 cups sugar)
   1 egg, well beaten
   1 tablespoon vanilla

Pour evaporated milk into freezer tray; freeze until ice
crystals form around edges. Chill beaters and bowl for
whipping. Soften gelatine in cold water. Scald milk. Combine flour, salt, and ¾ teaspoon sweetener; add enough additional cold water to make a smooth paste; add scalded
milk slowly. Cook 10 minutes over hot water, stirring often.
Add slowly to beaten egg. Cook and stir over hot (not
boiling) water until mixture coats spoon. Add softened gelatine; stir until dissolved. Remove from heat; add vanilla;
cool. Add remaining ¼ teaspoon sweetener to chilled
evaporated milk; whip until peaks form; fold into cooked
mixture; pour into freezing trays; place in freezer compart-
ment. After 30 minutes remove from tray to chilled bowl
and beat well. Repeat 3 times more, at half-hour intervals.
Freeze until firm. Makes about 1 quart. (*Calorie Savings:
approximately 1728*)

Paoli's Restaurant, San Francisco, California

LEMON SPONGE PIE OR PUDDING

    1 tablespoon soft butter or
      margarine
      Grated peel of 1 lemon
    ½ teaspoon liquid concentrated sweetener
      (= 1 cup sugar)
    3 eggs, separated
    2 tablespoons flour
    1 cup milk
    5 tablespoons lemon juice

Combine butter, lemon peel, sweetener, egg yolks, flour, and milk; beat well. Stir in lemon juice. Beat egg whites stiff; fold in.
1. Pour into 8-inch, baked pie shell. Bake at 375° for about 30 minutes or until puffed and golden brown

or

2. Pour into 5 or 6 custard cups. Set cups in pan of warm water. Bake at 350° for 40 to 45 minutes or until puffed and golden brown. (*Calorie Savings: approximately 864*)

Rudi's Club, Houston, Texas

* BE SURE TO CHECK YOUR BRAND OF SWEETENER'S SUGAR EQUIVALENT.

APPLE PIE

Pastry for 2-crust, 9-inch pie
6 *cups thinly sliced apples*
3 *tablespoons cold water*
1 *tablespoon cornstarch*
½ *teaspoon liquid concentrated sweetener*
  (= 1 cup sugar)
⅛ *teaspoon salt*
¼ *teaspoon nutmeg*
1 *teaspoon cinnamon*
2 *tablespoons butter or margarine*

Line piepan with pastry; fill pan with sliced apples. Blend water and cornstarch; add sweetener, salt, and spices; mix well. Spoon evenly over apples. Dot with butter. Cover with top crust; seal edges; flute; cut slits in center. Bake at 425° for 15 minutes. Lower heat to 375°; bake 20 to 25 minutes longer, or until apples are tender. (*Calorie Savings: approximately 864*)

The Garden, Knoxville, Tennessee

DESSERT OMELET

 1 tablespoon butter or margarine
 1 cup peeled, diced apples
 ½ cup orange juice
 ½ cup diced orange segments
 ½ cup diced grapefruit segments
 1 teaspoon lemon juice
 2 tablespoons chopped toasted almonds
 ¼ teaspoon vanilla
 8 drops liquid concentrated sweetener
   (= 4 teaspoons sugar)
 4-egg French omelet

Melt butter; add diced apples; cook over moderate heat for 15 minutes. Add orange juice, diced orange and grapefruit segments, lemon juice, and almonds. Simmer 10 minutes, stirring often and mashing with a fork. Remove from heat; stir in vanilla and sweetener. Spread on surface of cooked omelet and roll up. Makes 2 to 3 servings. (*Calorie Savings: approximately 72*)

Chez La Combe, Dallas, Texas

* BE SURE TO CHECK YOUR BRAND
OF SWEETENER'S SUGAR EQUIVALENT.

SABAYON MARSALA

2 egg yolks, slightly beaten
1 tablespoon Marsala wine
10 drops liquid concentrated sweetener
  (= 5 teaspoons sugar)

Combine egg yolks and wine in top of small double boiler. Whip over hot (not boiling) water until it thickens to consistency of whipped cream. Remove from heat; stir in sweetener. Serve warm, in sherbet glasses, as a dessert. Makes 2 servings. (*Calorie Savings: approximately 90*)

Rive Gauche, Washington, D.C.

APPLE WHIP

5 egg whites
⅛ teaspoon liquid concentrated sweetener
  (= ¼ cup sugar)
3 eating apples
  Nutmeg
  Custard (see page 55)

Beat egg whites until stiff; beat in sweetener. Core and peel apples; grate into acidulated water to cover (1 teaspoon lemon juice to each cup water) stirring often to keep apples from darkening. Drain apples thoroughly; fold into beaten egg whites. Turn into serving dish; sprinkle with nutmeg; chill. Serve with Custard made with egg yolks. Makes 6 servings. (*Calorie Savings: approximately 216*)

SWEET-POTATO PIE

1½ cups mashed sweet potatoes
½ cup undiluted evaporated milk
½ teaspoon cinnamon
½ teaspoon nutmeg
½ teaspoon allspice
½ teaspoon salt
3 eggs, separated
2 tablespoons butter or margarine
1 tablespoon grated orange peel
¼ teaspoon liquid concentrated sweetener
   (= ½ cup sugar)
1 envelope unflavored gelatine
¼ cup cold water
1 baked 9-inch pie shell
1 cup Whipped Topping (see page 55)

Combine mashed sweet potatoes, milk, spices, salt, egg yolks, and butter; cook and stir over medium heat until thickened. Remove from heat; stir in orange peel and sweetener. Soften gelatine in cold water; dissolve over hot water; add to sweet-potato mixture; mix thoroughly. Chill until partially set. Beat egg whites stiff; fold in. Spoon into baked pie shell; chill until set. Swirl Whipped Topping over surface. (*Calorie Savings: approximately 432*)

Rainbow Inn, Lima, Illinois

* BE SURE TO CHECK YOUR BRAND
OF SWEETENER'S SUGAR EQUIVALENT.

NOODLE KUGEL

8 ounces medium noodles, cooked
2 apples
¼ cup seedless raisins
2 eggs
1 cup milk
1 tablespoon dietetic jelly (any flavor)
24 drops liquid concentrated sweetener
   (= ¼ cup sugar)
½ teaspoon cinnamon
½ teaspoon vanilla
½ teaspoon salt
1 tablespoon butter or margarine

Drain noodles thoroughly. Core apples; peel; slice thin; add to noodles with raisins; mix well. Turn into casserole. Combine eggs, milk, jelly, sweetener, cinnamon, vanilla, and salt. Beat to blend. Pour over noodle mixture. Dot with butter. Bake at 350° for 30 minutes. Makes 6 to 8 servings. (*Calorie Savings: approximately 216*)

The Park Lane, Buffalo, New York

CHOCOLATE PUDDING

3 tablespoons cornstarch
Few grains salt
3 tablespoons breakfast cocoa (*not instant*)
2 cups skim milk
¼ teaspoon liquid concentrated sweetener
   (= ½ cup sugar)
1 teaspoon vanilla

Combine cornstarch, salt, and cocoa. Add milk gradually; stir until well blended. Cook and stir over medium heat until smooth and thick. Remove from heat; stir in sweetener and vanilla. Makes 6 servings. (*Calorie Savings: approximately 432*)

The Garden, Knoxville, Tennessee

* BE SURE TO CHECK YOUR BRAND
OF SWEETENER'S SUGAR EQUIVALENT.

MOLDED MOCHA PUDDING

3 tablespoons breakfast cocoa (*not instant*)
2 teaspoons cornstarch
4 teaspoons instant coffee powder
2 cups water, divided
2 eggs, separated
1 envelope unflavored gelatine
½ teaspoon liquid concentrated sweetener
   (= 1 cup sugar)
1 teaspoon vanilla
⅛ teaspoon salt
   Whipped Topping (see page 55)

Combine cocoa, cornstarch, and coffee in top of double boiler. Add 1¾ cups water; mix well. Bring to boil over direct heat. Cook and stir 5 minutes. Remove from heat. Beat egg yolks; add a little of the cocoa mixture. Stir into remaining cocoa mixture; set over hot water; cook and stir 2 or 3 minutes. Soften gelatine in remaining ¼ cup cold water; stir into hot mixture. Stir in sweetener, vanilla, and salt. Chill until partially set. Beat egg whites stiff; fold in. Spoon into individual molds; cover surface with waxed paper. Chill until set. Makes 4 to 6 servings, depending on size of mold. Serve with Whipped Topping. (*Calorie Savings: approximately 864*)

Hayden House, Omaha Airport
Omaha, Nebraska

FLAMING CHOCOLATE SUNDAE

2 tablespoons butter or margarine
3 tablespoons Dutch process breakfast cocoa
½ cup dietetic chocolate syrup
12 drops liquid concentrated sweetener
    (= 2 tablespoons sugar)
1 tablespoon dry brandy
1 pint Vanilla Ice Cream (see page 68)

Melt butter in chafing dish; blend in cocoa. Add syrup gradually, beating until smooth. When sauce begins to bubble, remove pan from heat. Stir in sweetener and brandy. Ignite; spoon over ice cream. Makes 4 servings. (*Calorie Savings: approximately 108*)

Westport Room, A Fred Harvey Restaurant
Kansas City, Missouri

* BE SURE TO CHECK YOUR BRAND
OF SWEETENER'S SUGAR EQUIVALENT.

ORANGE CUSTARD SOUFFLE

4 eggs, separated
½ teaspoon liquid concentrated sweetener
    (= 1 cup sugar)
¼ teaspoon salt
1 medium orange, grated peel and juice

Beat egg yolks until thick and lemon-colored. Beat in sweetener and salt. Add grated orange peel and juice. Beat egg whites stiff; fold in. Turn into buttered 1-quart soufflé dish. Set dish in pan of hot water (water should reach at least halfway up the dish). Bake at 325° for about 45 minutes. Makes 6 servings. (*Calorie Savings: approximately 864*)

The Dogwood Room, Airport 77 Restaurant
Charlotte, North Carolina

GRAPE ICE SUPREME

1 cup unsweetened grape juice
½ cup crushed dietetic pineapple
    Juice of 2 lemons
1 cup water
2 tablespoons cream sherry
½ teaspoon liquid concentrated sweetener
    (= 1 cup sugar)

Combine all ingredients; mix well. Freeze in refrigerator tray to a mush. Remove from tray; beat; return to tray; freeze firm. Makes 4 servings. (*Calorie Savings: approximately 864*)

The Dogwood Room, Airport 77 Restaurant
Charlotte, North Carolina

PUMPKIN CUP CUSTARDS

    1 teaspoon liquid concentrated sweetener
      (= 2 cups sugar)
    1½ cups skim milk
    1½ cups canned pumpkin
    2 eggs, slightly beaten
    ½ teaspoon vanilla
    ½ teaspoon cinnamon
    ¼ teaspoon powdered ginger
    ¼ teaspoon powdered cloves
    ¼ teaspoon mace
    ¼ teaspoon allspice
    ¼ teaspoon salt
    2 tablespoons butter or margarine, melted

Add sweetener to milk; stir well. Combine remaining ingredients; mix well. Add milk mixture slowly to pumpkin mixture while stirring. Pour into greased custard cups; set cups in pan of warm water. Bake at 350° for 45 minutes or until knife inserted near rim comes out clean. Chill. Makes 6 to 8 servings, depending on size of cups used. (*Calorie Savings: approximately 1728*)

Anderton's Restaurants, Memphis, Tennessee

* BE SURE TO CHECK YOUR BRAND
OF SWEETENER'S SUGAR EQUIVALENT.

ORANGE BRAN COOKIES

2 cups sifted all-purpose flour
1 teaspoon baking powder
¼ teaspoon salt
1 cup bran flakes
½ cup soft butter or margarine
1 egg
2 tablespoons orange juice
1 teaspoon grated orange peel
½ teaspoon lemon extract
1 teaspoon liquid concentrated sweetener
   (= 2 cups sugar)

Mix and sift flour, baking powder, and salt. Add remaining ingredients; beat until well blended. Form into 2 rolls 1½ inches in diameter; wrap in aluminum foil. Chill several hours or overnight. Slice thin. Place on greased baking sheets. Bake at 400° for 8 to 12 minutes. Makes about 6 dozen cookies. (*Calorie Savings: approximately 1728*)

Grison's Steak House, San Francisco, California

COFFEE ALMOND CUSTARD

1 quart milk
6 eggs, beaten smooth
1 tablespoon vanilla
1 tablespoon instant coffee powder
1 teaspoon liquid concentrated sweetener
    (= 2 cups sugar)
¼ cup canned, toasted slivered almonds

Scald milk. Combine eggs, vanilla, instant coffee, and sweetener. Pour hot milk slowly on egg mixture. Stir until well blended. Pour into 1½-quart casserole; set in pan of warm water. Bake at 325° for about 1 hour, or until knife inserted near edge comes out clean. Sprinkle with almonds. Chill. Makes 8 to 10 servings. (*Calorie Savings: approximately 1728*)

The Pontchartrain Hotel, New Orleans, Louisiana

ZABAGLIONE

6 eggs, separated
3 tablespoons cream sherry
½ teaspoon liquid concentrated sweetener
    (= 1 cup sugar)

Beat egg yolks slightly in top of double boiler. Add sherry. Beat over hot (not boiling) water until slightly thickened. Remove from heat. Stir in sweetener. Beat egg whites stiff but not dry; fold in. Spoon into serving dishes. Serve warm or chilled. Makes 6 servings. (*Calorie Savings: approximately 864*)

University Club, San Antonio, Texas

* BE SURE TO CHECK YOUR BRAND
OF SWEETENER'S SUGAR EQUIVALENT.

SHERRY BANANAS

4 *bananas*
1 *tablespoon lemon juice*
¼ *teaspoon ground cloves*
½ *cup cream sherry*
3 *tablespoons melted butter or margarine*
14 *drops liquid concentrated sweetener*
   (= *7 teaspoons sugar*)

Peel bananas; halve lengthwise; place in shallow baking dish. Combine remaining ingredients; pour over bananas. Broil, with surface of food 4 inches below heat, until golden brown, basting often with wine mixture. (*Calorie Savings: approximately 126*)

Kenny's Steak Pub, New York, New York

LIME CHIFFON PIE

1 egg
⅛ teaspoon salt
½ cup milk
1 cup water, divided
¾ teaspoon liquid concentrated sweetener
  (= 1½ cups sugar)
1 envelope unflavored gelatine
4 drops green food coloring
1 tablespoon grated lime peel
¼ cup lime juice
⅔ cup evaporated milk
1 baked 8-inch pie shell

Beat egg; add salt, milk, and ½ cup water. Cook and stir over hot (not boiling) water until mixture thickens; remove from heat; stir in sweetener. Soften gelatine in remaining cold water; add to hot-milk mixture; stir until dissolved. Stir in food coloring, lime peel, and lime juice. Chill until slightly thickened. Meanwhile, chill evaporated milk in freezer tray until ice crystals form around edge. Whip until stiff. Whip chilled gelatine mixture; fold into whipped evaporated milk. Spoon into baked pie shell. Chill until firm. (*Calorie Savings: approximately 1296*)

Tubbert's Restaurant, Syracuse, New York

* BE SURE TO CHECK YOUR BRAND
OF SWEETENER'S SUGAR EQUIVALENT.

[83]

FRESH APPLE CAKE

1¼ cups sifted all-purpose flour
2 teaspoons baking soda
1 teaspoon cinnamon
¼ teaspoon nutmeg
½ teaspoon salt
½ cup soft butter or margarine
1 teaspoon vanilla
1 egg
½ teaspoon liquid concentrated sweetener
  (= 1 cup sugar)
2 cups freshly grated apples
½ cup broken walnut meats

Mix and sift flour, baking soda, spices, and salt. Add butter, vanilla, egg, and sweetener; beat until well blended. Stir in grated apples and nuts. Turn into well-greased, 8-inch-square pan. Bake at 375° for 40 to 45 minutes. Cut in squares to serve. Makes 9 servings. (*Calorie Savings: approximately 864*)

Note: This is a moist cake. Excellent served warm with Lemon Sauce for Puddings (see *Contents*) as a cottage-pudding type of dessert.

House of Shish Kebab, Sacramento, California

SOODLY
(Armenian Rice Pudding)

1½ *quarts milk (6 cups)*
½ *cup raw, regular rice*
½ *teaspoon salt*
2 *eggs*
1 *teaspoon vanilla*
½ *teaspoon liquid concentrated sweetener*
   (= 1 *cup sugar*)
   Cinnamon or nutmeg

Combine milk, rice, and salt in heavy 2-quart saucepan; simmer 1 hour, stirring occasionally. Combine eggs, vanilla, and sweetener; beat well; add to rice mixture; cook and stir 1 minute. Pour into serving dish; sprinkle with cinnamon or nutmeg. Chill. Makes 8 servings. (*Calorie Savings: approximately 864*)

House of Shish Kebab, Sacramento, California

* BE SURE TO CHECK YOUR BRAND
OF SWEETENER'S SUGAR EQUIVALENT.

BANANAS RON RICO

6 *bananas*
Flour
¼ *cup butter or margarine*
4 *egg yolks*
1 *teaspoon cornstarch*
1 *teaspoon cinnamon*
2 *cups milk*
½ *teaspoon liquid concentrated sweetener*
  (= 1 cup sugar)
¼ *cup rum*

Peel bananas; cut in half lengthwise; dust with flour; sauté in butter or margarine until golden brown; remove to warm platter. Combine egg yolks, cornstarch, and cinnamon; beat until well blended. Add milk. Cook and stir over hot (not boiling) water until slightly thickened. Remove from heat; stir in sweetener and rum. Pour over bananas. Makes 6 servings. (*Calorie Savings: approximately 864*)

The Pontchartrain Hotel, New Orleans, Louisiana

LEMON CAKE-CUSTARD

   3 *large eggs, separated*
 ¼ *teaspoon salt*
 ¾ *teaspoon liquid concentrated sweetener*
   (= 1½ cups sugar)
 ⅓ *cup lemon juice*
   2 *tablespoons melted butter or margarine*
1½ *cups skim milk*
   5 *tablespoons flour*

Beat egg whites until soft peaks form. Add salt and sweetener; beat until stiff and glossy. Beat egg yolks slightly; add lemon juice, melted butter, and milk. Add egg-yolk mixture to flour slowly; beat until smooth. Fold in egg-white mixture. Pour into greased 1-quart casserole. Set casserole in pan of warm water. Bake at 350° for 1 hour 10 minutes. Makes 6 to 8 servings. (*Calorie Savings: approximately 1296*)

Anderton's Restaurants, Memphis, Tennessee

* BE SURE TO CHECK YOUR BRAND
OF SWEETENER'S SUGAR EQUIVALENT.

SPICY PUMPKIN PIE

¼ teaspoon mace
½ teaspoon allspice
1 teaspoon cinnamon
1 can (1 pound) pumpkin
½ teaspoon liquid concentrated sweetener
  (= 1 cup sugar)
1 cup skim milk
¼ cup browned butter
1 unbaked 9-inch pie shell

Stir spices into pumpkin; mix well. Stir in sweetener, milk, and browned butter. Pour into unbaked pie shell. Bake at 425° for 15 minutes. Lower heat to 350°; bake 45 minutes longer. (*Calorie Savings: approximately 864*)

Cross Keys Restaurant, Fort Worth, Texas

PEACHES FLAMBE

2 fresh peaches, sliced or
1 can dietetic peaches, drained
¾ cup orange juice
4 drops liquid concentrated sweetener
  (= 2 teaspoons sugar)
3 tablespoons brandy
Vanilla Ice Cream (see page 68)

Combine peaches, orange juice, and sweetener in chafing dish; bring to a boil. Warm brandy; pour over all; ignite. Serve, flaming, over Vanilla Ice Cream. Makes 4 servings. (*Calorie Savings: approximately 36*)

Westport Room, Kansas City, Missouri

PAPAYA JUBILEE FLAMBE

2 cups water
¼ teaspoon liquid concentrated sweetener
 (= ½ cup sugar)
1 tablespoon lemon juice
1 tablespoon cornstarch
2 tablespoons brandy
2 tablespoons port wine
1 papaya (about 4 pounds)
4 tablespoons 160-proof rum or brandy
 Vanilla Ice Cream (see page 68)

Bring water to boil. Remove from heat; add sweetener and lemon juice. Blend cornstarch with brandy and wine; add; cook over low heat, stirring, until slightly thickened. Continue cooking 10 minutes or until syrup is clear, stirring frequently. Peel papaya; remove seeds; cube; pour into large skillet. Add syrup. Cook just long enough to heat through. (Overcooking breaks down the papaya.) Pour into chafing dish. Pour 160-proof liquor evenly over all. Ignite. Spoon over Vanilla Ice Cream while flaming. Makes 8 servings. (*Calorie Savings: approximately 432*)

Westward Ho Hotel, Phoenix, Arizona

* BE SURE TO CHECK YOUR BRAND
OF SWEETENER'S SUGAR EQUIVALENT.

CHOCOLATE SPONGE PUDDING

2 *cups milk*
2 *squares unsweetened chocolate*
½ *teaspoon liquid concentrated sweetener*
   (= *1 cup sugar*)
4 *tablespoons flour*
¼ *teaspoon salt*
2 *tablespoons melted butter or margarine*
3 *eggs, separated*
1½ *teaspoons vanilla*

Heat milk and chocolate over hot water until chocolate is melted. Remove from heat; blend well with rotary beater. Add sweetener. Combine flour and salt in mixing bowl. Stir in melted butter. Beat egg yolks slightly; stir in with vanilla. Add milk mixture. Beat egg whites until they form soft peaks; fold in. Turn into greased 1-quart casserole; set in shallow pan. Pour warm water into pan to depth of 1 inch. Bake at 325° for 1 hour, or until knife inserted near rim comes out clean. Serve with sweetened cream (2 drops sweetener to 1 cup cream). Makes 8 servings. (*Calorie Savings: approximately 864*)

Ramon's, Denver, Colorado

BANANA CREAM PIE

    3 eggs, separated
    ½ cup skim milk
    ½ cup water
    1 envelope unflavored gelatine
    1 teaspoon vanilla
    ¼ teaspoon liquid concentrated sweetener
        (= ½ cup sugar)
    1 baked 9-inch pie shell
    1 medium-size banana, peeled and sliced thin

Beat egg yolks with milk and water until blended in top of double boiler; stir in gelatine. Cook, stirring constantly, over hot, not boiling, water 7 minutes, or until gelatine dissolves and mixture coats spoon; remove from heat. Stir in vanilla and sweetener. Chill 30 minutes, or until as thick as unbeaten egg white. Beat egg whites until they form soft peaks. Gradually fold in thickened gelatine mixture. Spoon filling into cooled pastry shell. Chill several hours, or until firm. When ready to serve, top with a ring of banana slices. (*Calorie Savings: approximately 432*)

Connoisseur Restaurant, Wichita, Kansas

* BE SURE TO CHECK YOUR BRAND
OF SWEETENER'S SUGAR EQUIVALENT.

[91]

CARIOCA FLUFF

1 envelope unflavored gelatine
2 cups skim milk
1 square unsweetened chocolate
⅛ teaspoon cinnamon
6 drops liquid concentrated sweetener
    (= 1 tablespoon sugar)
¼ teaspoon vanilla

Soften gelatine in milk in top of double boiler; stir in chocolate and cinnamon. Heat over boiling water, stirring often, until chocolate melts and gelatine dissolves; remove from heat. Add sweetener; stir in vanilla. Chill 1 hour, or until as thick as unbeaten egg whites. Set top of double boiler in a pan of ice and water; beat mixture until fluffy, light and double in volume. Spoon into 6 small molds or custard cups. Chill until firm. Unmold on dessert plates. (*Calorie Savings: approximately 54*)

Louisiane Restaurant, Tulsa, Oklahoma

ALMOND MERINGUE DROPS

    3 egg whites
  ¼ teaspoon cream of tartar
  32 drops liquid concentrated sweetener
       (= 16 teaspoons sugar)
    3 cups oven-popped rice cereal
  ¼ cup blanched almonds, chopped

Beat egg whites, cream of tartar, and sweetener until meringue forms soft peaks. Fold in cereal and almonds. Drop by rounded teaspoonfuls onto lightly greased cookie sheets. Bake at 350° for 15 minutes, or until lightly browned. Remove at once from cookie sheets; cool on wire racks. Makes 3 dozen. (*Calorie Savings: approximately 288*)

                              The Cloud Room, Airport Terminal
                                          Des Moines, Iowa

                    * BE SURE TO CHECK YOUR BRAND
              OF SWEETENER'S SUGAR EQUIVALENT.

SURPRISE CHEESECAKE

    2 eggs, separated
    1 cup water
    ¼ teaspoon salt
    ½ teaspoon liquid concentrated sweetener
      (= 1 cup sugar)
    2 envelopes unflavored gelatine
    ⅓ cup instant nonfat dry milk
    1 teaspoon grated lemon peel
    3 tablespoons lemon juice, divided
    1 teaspoon vanilla
    3 cups (1½ pounds) cream-style cottage cheese
    1 cup evaporated milk, well chilled

Beat egg yolks slightly; beat in water, salt, and sweetener.
Mix gelatine and dry milk in top of double boiler; stir in
egg-yolk mixture. Cook over simmering water, stirring constantly, about 5 minutes, or until gelatine dissolves and mixture coats spoon. Strain into large bowl; stir in lemon peel,
2 tablespoons lemon juice, and vanilla. Chill 30 minutes,
or until mixture is as thick as unbeaten egg whites. Press
cottage cheese through sieve; stir into gelatine mixture until
blended. Beat egg whites until they stand in firm peaks.
Beat chilled evaporated milk with remaining lemon juice
until stiff. Fold beaten egg whites, then whipped milk into
cheese mixture; pour into 8-cup mold; chill at least 4 hours,
or until softly set. Unmold onto serving plate. Slice into
wedge-shape pieces. (If desired, garnish with a ring of fresh
berries or sliced fresh fruit.) Makes 10 servings. (*Calorie
Savings: approximately 864*)

Fan and Bill's Restaurant, Atlanta, Georgia

PINEAPPLE SHERBET IN ORANGE CUPS

    2 cups buttermilk
    1 can (6 ounces) frozen concentrated pineapple
       juice, thawed
    ½ teaspoon liquid concentrated sweetener
       (= 1 cup sugar)
    6 small oranges, peeled
    6 whole strawberries, washed and hulled

Combine buttermilk and pineapple juice; add sweetener; beat until well blended. Pour into ice-cube tray, or 8-inch-square pan; freeze until firm almost to middle. Spoon into chilled bowl; beat quickly until fluffy-smooth; return to tray; freeze 2 to 3 hours longer, or until firm. Separate sections of each orange slightly to form a cup; place in dessert dishes; scoop sherbet into middle; garnish each with strawberry. Makes 6 servings. (*Calorie Savings: approximately 864*)

Louisiane Restaurant, Tulsa, Oklahoma

* BE SURE TO CHECK YOUR BRAND
OF SWEETENER'S SUGAR EQUIVALENT.

SCANDINAVIAN PRUNE PUDDING

2 cups prunes
½ cup prune liquid
⅛ teaspoon salt
¼ teaspoon cinnamon
⅛ teaspoon allspice
⅛ teaspoon nutmeg
1 cup boiling water
3 tablespoons cornstarch
⅓ cup cold water
¼ teaspoon plus 24 drops liquid concentrated
    sweetener
    (= ¾ cup sugar)
2 tablespoons lemon juice

Simmer prunes for 10 minutes in enough water to cover.
Cool. Drain; reserve liquid. Remove pits from prunes. Run
pulp through food mill or sieve. Add prune liquid, salt,
spices, and boiling water. Simmer 5 minutes. Blend cornstarch with cold water until smooth; add. Cook and stir
until thick. Simmer 10 minutes longer. Remove from heat.
Add sweetener and lemon juice. Chill. Serve with plain or
whipped cream, if desired. Makes 6 servings. (*Calorie Savings: approximately 648*)

Trinkaus Manor, Oriskany, New York

ORANGE CUSTARD

4 *oranges*
30 *drops liquid concentrated sweetener*
    (= 5 tablespoons sugar)
4 *eggs*
    Few grains salt
    Whipped Topping (see page 55)

Squeeze oranges; remove all white from peel; cut up orange part of peel; add to juice. Bring to a boil; remove from heat; let stand 2 hours; strain; discard peel; bring to boil again. Remove from heat; stir in sweetener. Beat eggs with salt; add hot orange juice mixture slowly to eggs. Cook and stir over hot (not boiling) water until thickened. Pour into *pot de crème* dishes or custard cups; chill. Garnish with Whipped Topping and, if desired, grated orange peel. Makes 6 servings. (*Calorie Savings: approximately 270*)

Rive Gauche, Washington, D.C.

* BE SURE TO CHECK YOUR BRAND
OF SWEETENER'S SUGAR EQUIVALENT.

[97]

JELLIED COFFEE SOUFFLE

1½ tablespoons unflavored gelatine
1¼ cups strong cold coffee, divided
 1 cup milk
 2 eggs, separated
 ⅛ teaspoon salt
 ¼ teaspoon vanilla
 ¼ teaspoon liquid concentrated sweetener
    (= ½ cup sugar)

Soften gelatine in ½ cup cold coffee. Combine remaining coffee and milk in top of double boiler. Beat egg yolks with salt; add to coffee mixture; cook and stir until slightly thickened; add softened gelatine; cook and stir a few minutes longer until gelatine dissolves. Remove from heat; add vanilla and sweetener; chill until slightly thickened. Beat egg whites stiff; fold in. Spoon into custard cups or individual molds; chill until firm. Makes 6 to 8 servings. (*Calorie Savings: approximately 432*)

The Garden Seat, Clearwater, Florida

MICHELLE'S DELIGHT

    4 eggs
    1 teaspoon lemon juice
   15 drops liquid concentrated sweetener
      (= 7½ teaspoons sugar)
    2 cups Whipped Topping, divided (see page 55)
    3 bananas
    2 tablespoons chopped toasted almonds

Whip eggs and lemon juice until thick and light. Cook and
stir over hot (not boiling) water about 5 minutes. Stir in
sweetener; remove from heat; cool. Fold in half the
Whipped Topping. Slice bananas into 6 dessert glasses;
cover with sauce; garnish with remaining topping; scatter
almonds on top; chill. Makes 6 servings. (*Calorie Savings:
approximately 135*)

Chez La Combe, Dallas, Texas

* BE SURE TO CHECK YOUR BRAND
OF SWEETENER'S SUGAR EQUIVALENT.

FRENCH CREOLE PUDDING

1¼ cups sifted all-purpose flour
2 teaspoons baking powder
⅛ teaspoon salt
¼ cup soft shortening
1 egg
¼ teaspoon liquid concentrated sweetener
     (= ½ cup sugar)
½ cup milk
1 can (1 pound) dietetic apricots

Mix and sift flour, baking powder, and salt. Add shortening, egg, sweetener, and milk; beat well until mixture forms a smooth batter. Heat apricots with their juice to boiling point; pour into 1-quart casserole. Pour batter evenly over fruit. Bake at 350° for 45 minutes. Turn out, upside down, on serving dish. If desired, serve with sherry-flavored whipped cream. Makes 6 servings. (*Calorie Savings: approximately 432*)

Jack Sabin's Restaurant, Baton Rouge, Louisiana

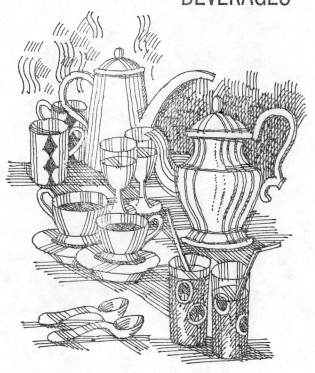

ZABERERS WHISKY SOUR

⅓ cup orange juice
2 tablespoons lemon juice
2 tablespoons rye whisky
5 drops liquid concentrated sweetener
    (= 2½ teaspoons sugar)

Measure ingredients into shaker. Add shaved ice; shake well. Pour into sour glass. Serves 1. (*Calorie Savings: approximately 45*)

O'ZABERERS IRISH COFFEE

¾ cup strong, hot coffee
2 tablespoons Irish whisky
4 drops liquid concentrated sweetener
    (= 2 teaspoons sugar)
Whipped cream

Pour coffee into 8-ounce tumbler. Add whisky and sweetener; stir well. Top with whipped cream. Drink through the cream. Serves 1. (*Calorie Savings: approximately 36*)

Zaberers Old Gable Inn, May's Landing, New Jersey

* BE SURE TO CHECK YOUR BRAND
OF SWEETENER'S SUGAR EQUIVALENT.

SABIN'S SWEET-NOG

    6 eggs
   16 drops liquid concentrated sweetener
       (= 8 teaspoons sugar)
   ¼ teaspoon cinnamon
   ¼ teaspoon ginger
   ¼ teaspoon ground cloves
    2 quarts chilled orange juice
   ½ cup lemon juice
    1 quart Vanilla Ice Cream (see page 68)
    1 quart sugar-free ginger ale
      Nutmeg

Beat eggs until thick and lemon-colored; beat in sweetener
and spices. Stir in orange and lemon juices. Just before
serving cut Vanilla Ice Cream in small cubes; put into
punch bowl. Pour juice mixture and ginger ale over ice
cream. Sprinkle with nutmeg. Makes about 24 punch-cup
servings. (*Calorie Savings: approximately 116*)

Jack Sabin's Restaurant, Baton Rouge, Louisiana

CAFE BRULOT

    Peel of 2 lemons
    Peel of 2 oranges
20 whole cloves (about)
 2 sticks cinnamon (2 inches each)
¾ cup dry brandy
 2 tablespoons apricot brandy
 5 drops liquid concentrated sweetener
    (= 2½ teaspoons sugar)
 1 quart strong hot coffee

Remove peel in sections from lemons and oranges; stick a
whole clove in each section of peel. Place in chafing dish.
Break cinnamon sticks in half; add. Combine dry brandy,
apricot brandy, and sweetener; stir well; pour into chafing
dish. Warm slightly; ignite. Pour in coffee slowly. Serve in
demitasses. Makes about 12 servings. (*Calorie Savings:
approximately 45*)

Brennan's, New Orleans, Louisiana

* BE SURE TO CHECK YOUR BRAND
OF SWEETENER'S SUGAR EQUIVALENT.

[105]

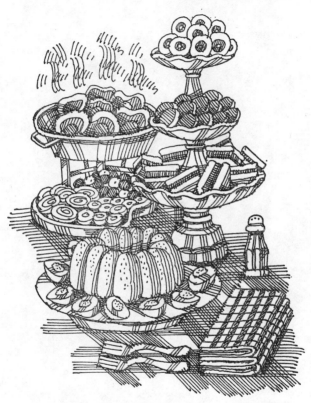

COLD BORSCHT

1 can (1 pound) shredded beets
4 cups water
3 tablespoons lemon juice
Salt to taste
15 drops liquid concentrated sweetener
   (= 7½ teaspoons sugar)
2 eggs, well beaten
Dairy sour cream

Combine beets with their liquid, water, lemon juice, and salt. Simmer 45 minutes. Remove from heat; stir in sweetener. Pour slowly into beaten eggs, stirring rapidly. Chill about 6 hours. Top each serving with a dollop of sour cream. Makes 6 servings. (*Calorie Savings: approximately 153*)

SOUTHERN CORN CAKE

¾ cup corn meal
1 cup flour
12 drops liquid concentrated sweetener
   (= 2 tablespoons sugar)
5 teaspoons baking powder
¾ teaspoon salt
1 cup milk
1 egg, well beaten
2 tablespoons vegetable oil

Mix and sift dry ingredients; add remaining ingredients; stir just enough to mix. Turn into shallow, greased pan. Bake at 425° for 20 minutes. Makes 6 servings. (*Calorie Savings: approximately 108*)

* BE SURE TO CHECK YOUR BRAND
OF SWEETENER'S SUGAR EQUIVALENT.

SPICY APPLE PANCAKES

        2 *cups buttermilk pancake mix*
    1 ¾ *cups skim milk*
        1 *egg*
        2 *tablespoons vegetable oil*
        1 *tablespoon lemon juice*
       ¼ *teaspoon liquid concentrated sweetener*
          (= ½ *cup sugar*)
       ¾ *teaspoon cinnamon*
        1 *apple*

Combine all ingredients except apple; beat until smooth.
Pare and core apple; grate into batter; stir to mix. Bake on
hot griddle until puffed and bubbly; turn to cook other side.
Makes about 20 pancakes. (*Calorie Savings: approximately
432*)

Smith's Cross Lake Inn, Shreveport, Louisiana

SPOON BREAD

2½ cups milk
¾ cup white corn meal
½ teaspoon salt
12 drops liquid concentrated sweetener
   (= 2 tablespoons sugar)
2 tablespoons butter or margarine
3 eggs, separated

Scald milk; stir in corn meal and salt; cook and stir 5 minutes. Remove from heat; add sweetener and butter; stir until butter melts. Beat egg yolks slightly; blend with a little of the corn-meal mixture; return to remaining corn-meal mixture. Beat egg whites stiff; fold in. Bake at 350° for 45 minutes. Makes 6 servings. (*Calorie Savings: approximately 108*)

St. Anthony Hotel, San Antonio, Texas

* BE SURE TO CHECK YOUR BRAND
OF SWEETENER'S SUGAR EQUIVALENT.

ONION SOUP

    6 cups thinly sliced white onions
    6 tablespoons butter or margarine
    2 pieces bay leaf
    1 tablespoon chopped parsley
    2 quarts hot water
    ¼ cup instant chicken-broth mix
    1 tablespoon Kitchen Bouquet
    1 tablespoon Worcestershire sauce
    5 drops liquid concentrated sweetener
      (= 2½ teaspoons sugar)
      Freshly ground black pepper
      Croutons
      Grated Parmesan cheese

Cook onions in butter until lightly browned. Add bay leaf, parsley, hot water, instant-broth mix, Kitchen Bouquet, and Worcestershire sauce. Bring to boil; lower heat; simmer about 1 hour, or until onions are tender. Add sweetener and pepper to taste. Top with croutons and grated cheese. Makes 6 to 8 servings. (*Calorie Savings: approximately 44*)

Casa Lorenzo, Syracuse, New York

CRANBERRY RELISH

3 *large navel oranges*
3 *large red apples*
1 *pound fresh cranberries*
1 *teaspoon liquid concentrated sweetener*
   (= 2 *cups sugar*)

Cut unpeeled oranges into chunks; remove any seeds. Core apples; do not peel; cut into eighths. Put oranges, apples, and cranberries through food chopper, using medium knife. Add sweetener; mix well. Makes about 5 cups. (*Calorie Savings: approximately 1728*)

Skoby's Restaurant, Kingsport, Tennessee

CINNAMON TOAST

4 *tablespoons soft butter or margarine*
30 *drops liquid concentrated sweetener*
   (= 5 *tablespoons sugar*)
1 *teaspoon cinnamon*
4 *slices bread*

Blend first 3 ingredients. Toast bread on one side. Spread untoasted side with butter mixture. Broil until browned. Cut toast into lengthwise strips or triangles. Makes 2 servings. (*Calorie Savings: approximately 270*)

University Club, San Antonio, Texas

* BE SURE TO CHECK YOUR BRAND
OF SWEETENER'S SUGAR EQUIVALENT.

CURRY DIP FOR SHRIMP

1 large onion, chopped (1 cup)
1 cup chicken broth, divided
1 tablespoon curry powder
¼ teaspoon salt
¼ teaspoon ground ginger
1 can (about 8 ounces) dietetic applesauce
8 drops liquid concentrated sweetener
  (= 4 teaspoons sugar)
2 teaspoons lemon juice

Cook onion slowly in ½ cup broth in small saucepan, stirring often, 10 minutes, or until onion is soft. Stir in curry powder; cook 1 minute; add salt, ginger, applesauce, sweetener, and remaining ½ cup broth; mix well. Simmer, stirring often, 5 minutes, or until thick. Just before serving, stir in lemon juice. Serve warm or chilled. Makes 1½ cups. (*Calorie Savings: approximately 72*)

Henry's, Cherry Hill, New Jersey

INDEX

[115]